FINISH FASTER!

20 Things to Remember Before Your
First or Your Next Marathon

EAMONN COFFEY

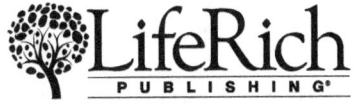

LifeRich Publishing is a registered trademark of The Reader's Digest Association, Inc.

LifeRich Publishing books may be ordered through booksellers or by contacting:

LifeRich Publishing
1663 Liberty Drive
Bloomington, IN 47403
www.liferichpublishing.com
844-686-9607

ISBN: 978-1-4897-3677-2 (sc)
ISBN: 978-1-4897-3678-9 (e)

Library of Congress Control Number: 2021913027

Print information available on the last page.

LifeRich Publishing rev. date: 07/20/2021

"The will to win means nothing
without the will to prepare."

Juma Ikangaa
– Tanzanian running champion and Boston Marathon winner.

CONTENTS

Guts

GEAR

#1 NEVER RUN IN BRAND NEW SHOES!

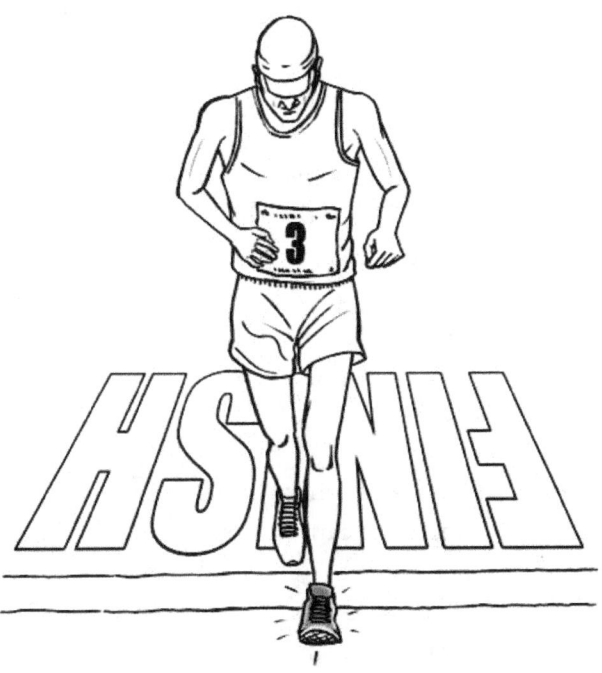

Even if you have never heard of Dick Beardsley until now it's interesting to know that he was an outstanding American marathon runner during the early '80s. He is best remembered for his "Duel

In The Sun" * with another great marathoner of that time – Alberto Salazar – at the 1982 Boston Marathon. Beardsley mildly injured his foot (which became a bigger problem later) while Salazar, the eventual winner, went to the hospital suffering from heatstroke.

Like any other great runner Dick Beardsley had to run some first marathons. One of those was The City Of Lakes Marathon (later merged with The Saint Paul Marathon to become the now well-known Twin Cities Marathon). The day before the race Dick visited a small race expo (nothing like today's huge extravaganzas) to get his race bib number. Ambling through some merchandising booths he saw an Adidas sign and headed to a table that displayed various types of running shoes. One pair of new bright white running shoes caught his eye. He liked them immediately and tried them on. They fit perfectly and felt amazingly comfortable. He decided to buy the shoes and run in them the next day.

As the race commenced the following morning Dick felt fine. This changed quickly though. By mile 5 his feet were becoming sore. At mile 10 all he could think of were his feet. Around Mile 15 he considered abandoning the race but persevered. At Mile 20 he looked down and realized his feet were bleeding. As he finished the race he looked down again to discover the beautiful white shoes had turned pink!

Lesson: Never run a marathon in Brand New Shoes! It's one of the most foolish things you can do. Instead race in shoes that are already broken in. If possible they should have, at least, 50 miles on them including, preferably, one long run to 20 miles. Conversely, don't run in shoes that are old and run down (with more than 500 miles run).

*Title of the excellent book about the event written by John Brandt.

#2 NEVER RUN IN BRAND NEW SOCKS!

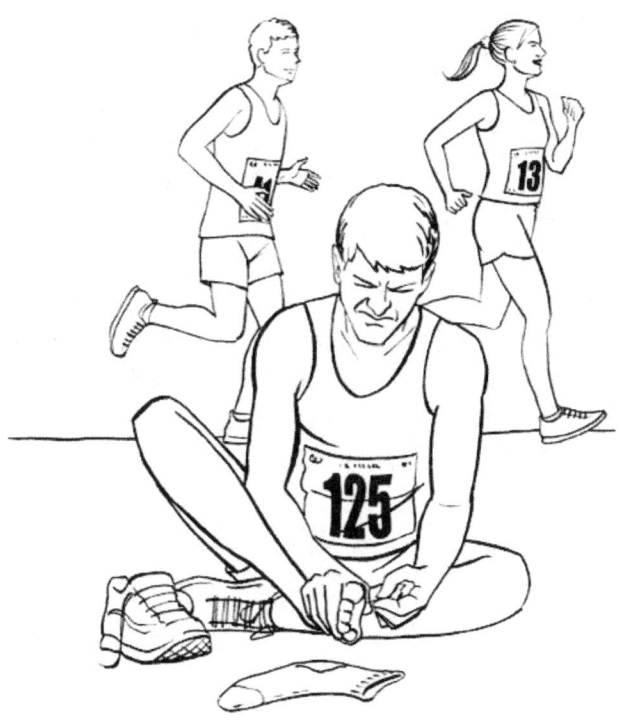

In 1988 I ran the Twin Cities Marathon in Minneapolis. It was a cold and blustery day with the temperature hovering around 42°F at the start. Because of the weather I decided to run in some comfortable warm socks I had purchased the previous day. This was my first time to do this after having run fifteen previous marathons in well-worn socks. Thinking back to Tip #1 I should have know better and why I did so I will never know.

After running the first half mile I began to notice the socks. By Mile 3 my right foot was starting to feel hot. By mile 5 there was a point in the middle of the sole of my right foot that was starting to bother me. By mile 10 that foot was shouting, no, screaming at me. I was forced to stop and take the shoe off and examine the foot. There was a large blister about the size of a quarter which contained fluid. I used one of my race bib pins to puncture the blister and drain the fluid. After getting back in the race I managed to finish in very reasonable time. Of course, I spend days afterward wondering how much better my race might have been if run in well-worn socks. I then wondered If I should have sent the new socks through the washer/dryer cycle at my hotel to make them softer and more broken-in for the race next day.

Lesson: Never run in brand new socks. It's almost as bad as running in brand new shoes as I found out to my regret. Instead run in socks you have run in previously and your feet are used to but be sure you will be comfortable in them beforehand.

#3 DOUBLE KNOT YOUR SHOELACES

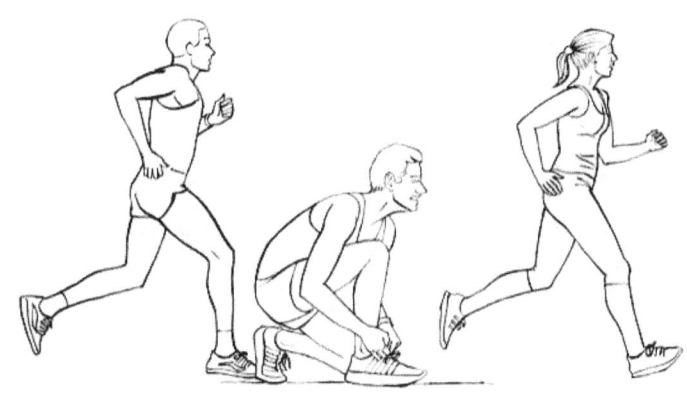

I was well prepared and ready to run a good marathon at LA III in sunny Los Angeles, California in 1988. I had done many long runs in practice in Minnesota and thought I could break three hours for the third time because of the flat course. I got off to a good, comfortable start and everything was going to plan until one of my shoelaces unraveled. I had to stop and quickly re-lace it. This affected my momentum and added unnecessary elapsed time into my race effort. After another three 3 miles or so it UNLACED

AGAIN! This time, recalling something a fellow runner had told me years before, I double-knotted both of my shoelaces and it was no longer a problem. While I ran a very acceptable 3:10:51 race time on a hot day I didn't break 3 hours and still wonder if I would have had I properly knotted my shoelaces beforehand.

Lesson: This may seem trivial but double knot your shoelaces before you start. This eliminates unnecessary time spent tying your laces in some part of the race. Remember you are not out to set a course record but you could get run into by another runner who doesn't see you as you squat down (especially after a crowded start or at a water stop). That could put you out of the race or, worse still, in the emergency room.

#4 TAKE OUT THE TRASH!

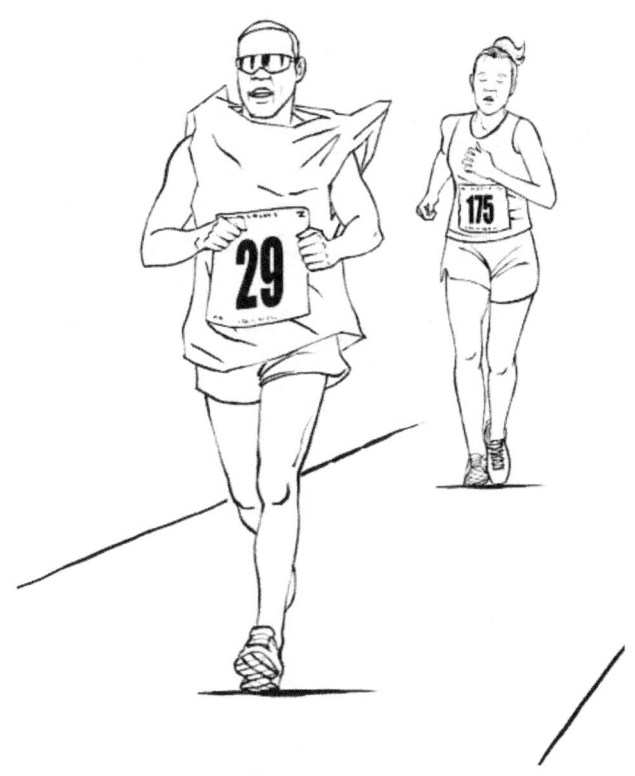

Since I ran many marathons in the Midwest or the East Coast I became very used to changing weather conditions and cooler temperatures at the starts of races. At first I used a light nylon parka but found this awkward and uncomfortable after a few miles. Then I switched to wearing two t-shirts. However, I soon found that I would invariably toss one t-shirt at some point in the race and had qualms about creating a refuse problem for someone else to clean up. Then during a mid-80s marathon I saw a runner wearing a trash bag for the first time and realized how great an idea this was. Any time after that if I thought the start was going to be cold I would bring along a trash bag with holes punched out for head and arms and wore it for the start of the race. Once I warmed up after a few miles I would take the trash bag off, fold it up as I raced along, and made it small enough to fit in the utility pocket of my running shorts. I then disposed of it properly after I'd finished the race.

Lesson: With average start temperatures of 60 degrees at many marathons, it's unlikely you'll be cold beforehand so don't overdress. After 10 miles your body acts like a mobile furnace and keeping it cool will be your biggest concern. If you want to avoid an early race chill, bring a trash bag to the start with holes for your head and arms. It's of negligible weight and you can discard it, properly, almost anywhere.

GRUB

#5 GO PASTA!

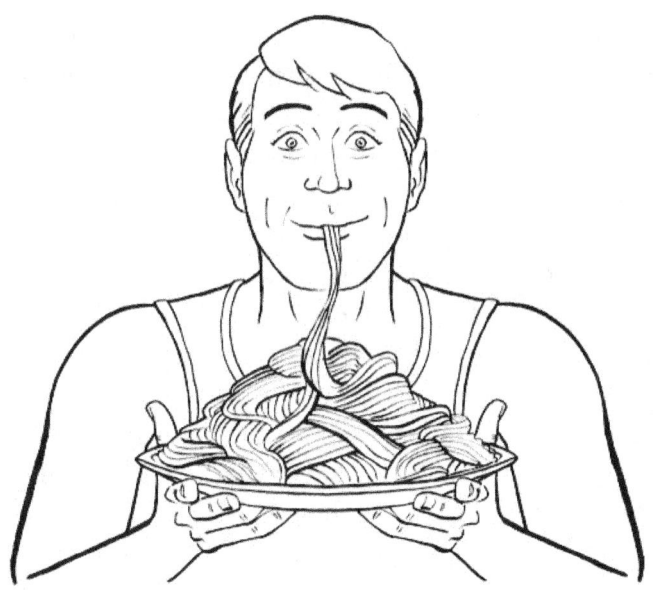

After running a half a dozen marathons and constantly looking for ways to get to the finish line faster other than running miles I decided to really exploit the whole concept of carbohydrate loading. Along with drinking lots of water throughout out the week, having a big pasta meal the night before the race is part of nearly every marathon preparation. The original thinking regarding carbo loading suggested that the runner should deplete his or her glycogen stores as much as possible by eating protein almost exclusively for a period of time. Then the runner ran what's called a "depletion run" to fully exhaust his or her remaining carbohydrate stores. After that, one simply reversed field and did nothing but eat pasta or other carbohydrate until race day to maximize glycogen storage.

I took this idea to an extreme. Seven days before the race I started eating protein at every meal. This was okay for about 48 hours. Since I was still running but much fewer miles I was working my way through the glycogen stores I had. On the fifth day before the race, I started to feel tight and sore. At this point I decided to do my depletion run. I hardly got through it and was totally exhausted afterwards. When I woke up the next morning, on Day Four, I felt like I had a hangover. Then I noticed my breath was starting to smell sweet. I checked around and found I had developed ketosis. That's to say I had developed a metabolic state characterized by elevated levels of ketone bodies in my blood and urine. Physiologic ketosis is a normal response to low glucose availability which comes from low carbohydrate diets and fasting. This provides an additional energy source for the brain in the form of ketones. That's why I thought I had a hangover. I seriously thought of abandoning my race. But as soon as I started to eat carbohydrate again things changed quickly. Within 24 hours I was back to normal and ran one of my better marathons on race day. After more study I discovered what I had done was over the top and unnecessary.

<u>Lesson</u>: In deciding to carbo load do the following: From day six to four before the race eat a <u>mixed diet</u> (not an exceptionally low carb/high protein diet as I did). Run a properly-paced depletion run on day four of 8 to 10 miles. Then eat as many carbohydrates as you reasonably can from day three to the race day. Don't overeat, just <u>increase the percentage</u> of carbohydrate in your normal meals.

#6 BUT DON'T OVERDO IT...

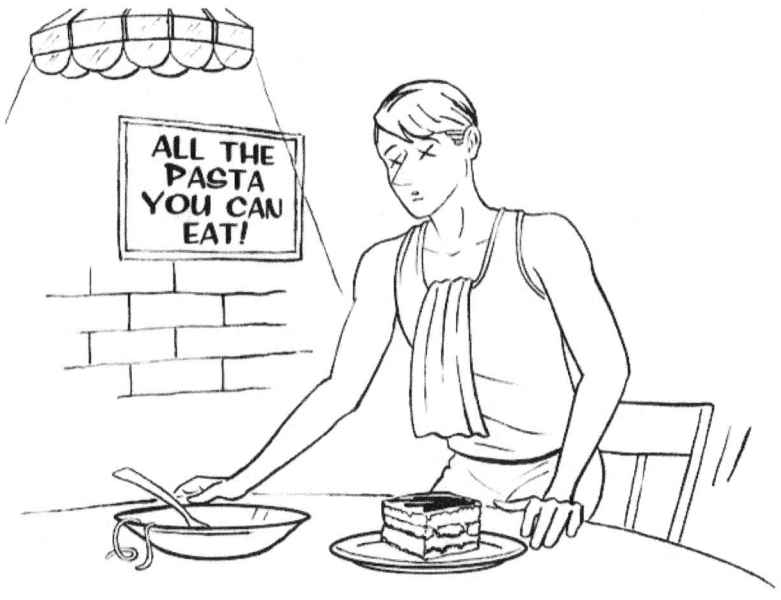

My first marathon ever was Grandmas Marathon in Duluth, Minnesota way back in 1982. I drove the 135 miles up from Minneapolis the day before and checked into one of the local hotels. Later I met some fellow runners I had done quite a bit of training with the weeks before in the Twin Cities. We found a nice Italian restaurant and started to carbo load on spaghetti. The restaurant had an "all you can eat" offer as an enticement to lure customers to their location. I think you know where this is going but to underscore what happened next you need to know that the restaurant offered a free dessert to anyone who could eat the most spaghetti at a table. Suffice to say I won the contest and waddled back to my room with Tiramisu under my arm to eat before I fell into bed. Despite a satisfactory visit to the bathroom before the race the next morning I felt like a stuffed goose until about ten miles into the race.

Lesson: It takes 16 to 18 hours for your body to process the carbohydrates you eat into glycogen, the fuel your running muscles need. Don't overeat the night before the race. Eat your last full meal 12 hours before the start of your race. This means you will get to the starting line and run the race on an empty colon (lower intestine) and won't have to visit the bathroom during the race. If you want to pig out, do it two nights before the race.

#7 WATER THE HORSE!

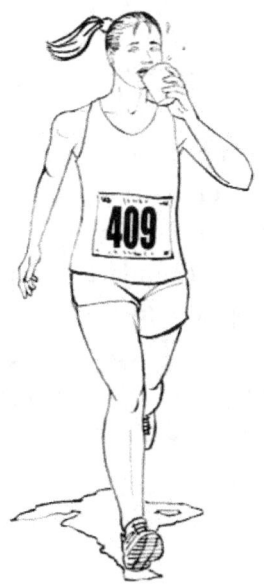

It's a strange thing but despite so much good modern advice to the contrary many runners still don't drink water until they absolutely must. In fact, from 1912 to 2001, the IAAF (International Amateur Athletic Federation) had a Rule Number 165:5 which stipulated that marathon runners could drink no fluids before the 11 kM mark (almost 7 miles) of a marathon and could only drink every 5 kM after that (the organization is now known as World Athletics). This was once true of the Boston Marathon also. I was part of that crowd for a while. I had the notion that the time I would "waste" at the water stop would not be made up for later. Then I ran a hotter than forecast marathon and learned a lesson. <u>You are dehydrated well before you feel thirsty</u>. After that I read everything I could find about water replacement in long distance running. One of the facts I discovered was that by the time you feel thirsty it's already too late. You will be drinking into a water deficit for the rest of your race. It is possible to drink too much water (the condition is called hyponatremia where sodium levels become dangerously low) but it's an extremely rare occurrence. Drinking water before and during your race is by far the best idea.

Lesson: It is physically impossible to replace all the fluid you will perspire during a marathon but you must do everything you can to help. Start drinking water from the very first aid station. Don't gulp, you can trap air in your stomach which can quickly give you a side stitch. Also don't stop dead in your tracks it could impede other runners and get you injured. Keep moving as you sip slowly over a period of time and distance. Try creasing the cup rim into a "V" on one side so you can sip and run at a decent pace until finishing all the water you can.

#8 UNCLOG THE COGS

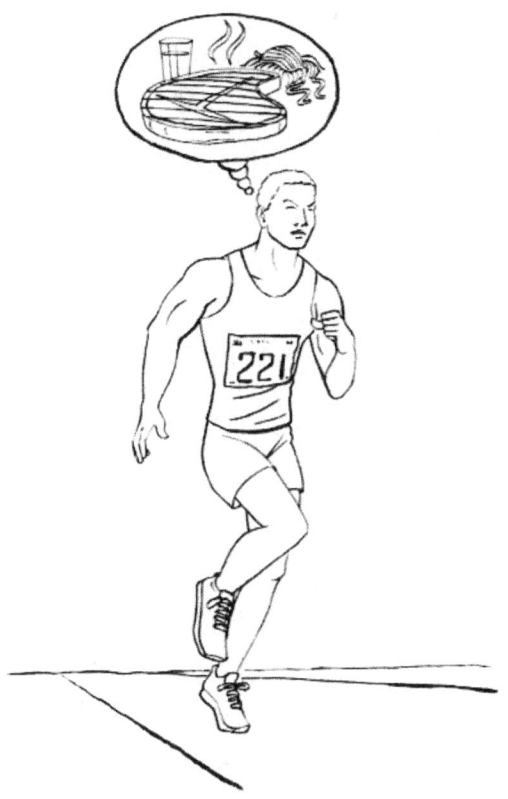

I have a friend named Bill. He's from Texas and a big meat eater. In fact, I think he eats meat just about every day of his life. He seems to think it's right up there with the flag and apple pie (which he eats a lot of too). He's a muscular guy and deserves his food there's no doubt. However, he does this kind of eating right up to marathon day except to replace the pie with spaghetti. I've tried a few times to explain to Bill the wisdom of backing off on red meat the week of the race but he won't hear of it. He gets this look on his face that as much says "You've got to be kidding". The sad thing is he's a surprisingly good runner despite all the muscles and would run much better times if he were more selective with his diet in the days leading up to his target race.

Lesson: Try to avoid eating red meat the week before the race. The high protein and saturated fat in it will tend to clog up your system and you will store less glycogen. Also, if possible, avoid drinking milk 24 – 48 hours before the race. It is a mucous-generating fluid and can clog up your nasal passages. You could be expectorating heavily for the first four or five miles of your race.

#9 COFFEE WORKS
BUT BE CAREFUL...

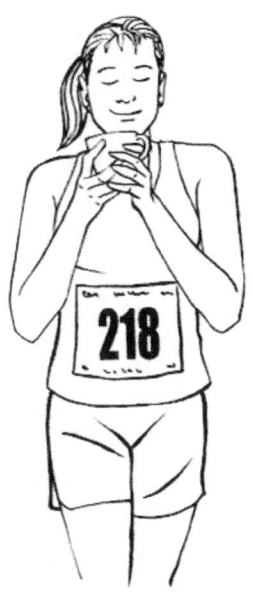

I ran eight Twin Cities Marathons in a row from the inaugural race in 1982 through 1989 before I left Minnesota and moved to California. Since I was always trying to improve my finish times this gave me a unique opportunity to try new things and make comparisons. One of those new things was drinking coffee before the race. As you should now be aware the reason some runners "hit the wall" and then "bonk" is because after 18 to 20 miles their bodies have run out of glycogen and must switch to fat as the next available energy source. For a trained runner with numerous long runs to 20 miles or more this will be much more comfortable than the untrained runner. This change can take some time and untrained runners will suffer in between. Coffee was said to speed up this change. I experimented with drinking coffee right before those Twin Cities Marathons and discovered that coffee did make a difference for me BUT there were drawbacks. First, the best dose appeared to be about 2 mg of caffeine per pound of body weight. That's 300 mgs of caffeine for the average 150-pound runner. That's two large cups of hot brewed coffee before you start this major race effort. It's a lot of fluid. If you drink the coffee too early it will become urine and you will have to expel it at some point during the race. That's what happened to me the first time out. I found I lost more time to pit-stops than I gained from the caffeine. I also found that if I could drink the coffee within 10 minutes of the start it would never become urine since as soon as I started running a lot of the blood in my body went to my legs. This shut off essential processes in my digestive system (such as making urine) and I would sweat the fluid off instead. I also discovered that if I could cool the coffee down to lukewarm I could chug the two cups with relative ease. The bottom line was I seemed to be able to improve my finish time by about 1%. Over a three hour marathon that's about 1 minute and 48 seconds which is a lot of time. I qualified for the Boston Marathon using this one idea.

Lesson: If you're a coffee drinker, drinking two cups of coffee within ten minutes of the race start can improve endurance and performance but it's a highly individual thing. It helps some but doesn't seem to help others. If you don't normally drink coffee, don't try it.

GUMPTION

#10 SLEEP IS WHERE YOU FIND IT

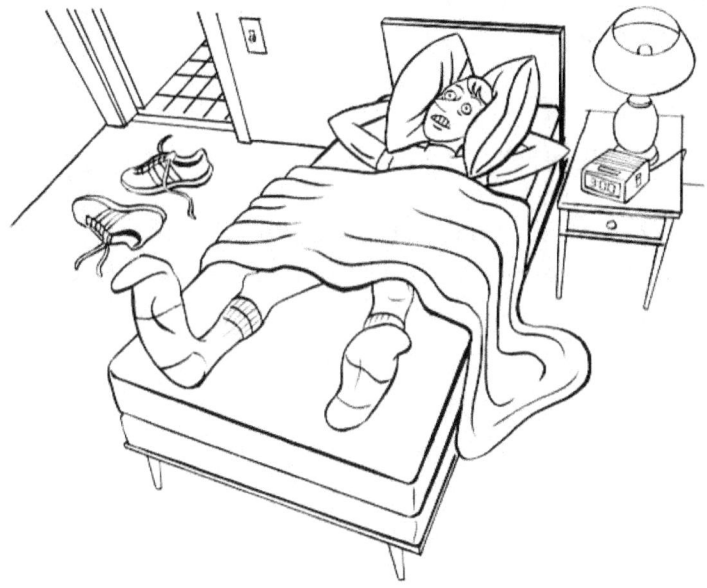

In 1998 I ran the Silicon Valley Marathon in San Jose, California. after traveling up the previous day on a bus from Irvine, California with a bunch of other runners from my then local running club. There was lots of distraction, commotion, and hijinks on the bus on the way up. In addition, we had a big "pasta feed" at a local restaurant after we arrived. I went to bed early thinking that the food would knock me out which it did - for a couple of hours. Because I had drunk a lot of water during the meal I woke up at about midnight to go to the bathroom and went back to bed again. I never slept another wink. Whether it was the long drive, the big meal or all the hoopla I will never know.

The next day, because of the lack of sleep, I started slowly and at about 10 miles picked up the pace confident I'd do okay since I'd gotten an excellent night's sleep two nights before the race. I kept that pace for the rest of the marathon and finished in 3:29:55 at almost exactly an 8:00 minute per mile pace. This was much better than I should have reasonably expected given the circumstances but the solid eight hours sleep two nights before really made a big difference.

Lesson: Make sure you get a good night's sleep two nights before the race. You may be too excited or distracted to sleep properly the night before the race, but that's all right once you've slept well the previous night. Furthermore, being rested also means taking it easy the day before the race. Minimize running or other time spent on one's feet.

#11 BE LIKE THE TORTOISE!

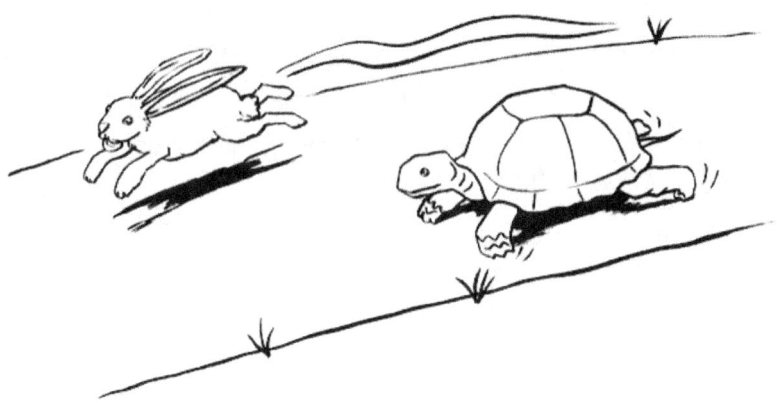

Remember the Aesop's fable about the tortoise the hare? That's the lesson to be thinking about as you start your race. You have just spent the last week prior to your race taking it easy and loading up on pasta to increase your glycogen levels. The typical 150-pound runner can store about 2,000 calories worth of glycogen. If you've done it right that should get you to about 20 miles at your planned pace depending on how efficient a runner you are. The worst thing you can do is start out too quickly. Think about your car. If you drive the average well-built sedan its best efficiency comes between

55-60 miles per hour. However, if you drive like you are the pace setter at the Indianapolis 500 the car's efficiency will go to pot. The same is true of your body. Start out slowly. If you do, your body will use up your glycogen stores slowly. While it's tempting to "bank" time early in the race don't overdo it. Avoid starting out too quickly as you will deplete a whole lot of glycogen unnecessarily and fade to gray (if not black – as in out of the race) too soon.

Instead start out slowly at your training pace plus one minute per mile (e.g., if your training pace is 7:00 per mile then start at 7:00 + 1:00 or 8:00 per mile pace). Then gradually pick up the pace as the race progresses until you are comfortably up to your goal pace in a reasonable amount of time.

Lesson: Don't start out too fast! You will deplete your glycogen stores too quickly and have real energy problems by mile 15. Also, starting out too fast will tire you out too quickly and may even give you side stitches by mile 5.

#12 IT'S YOUR RACE

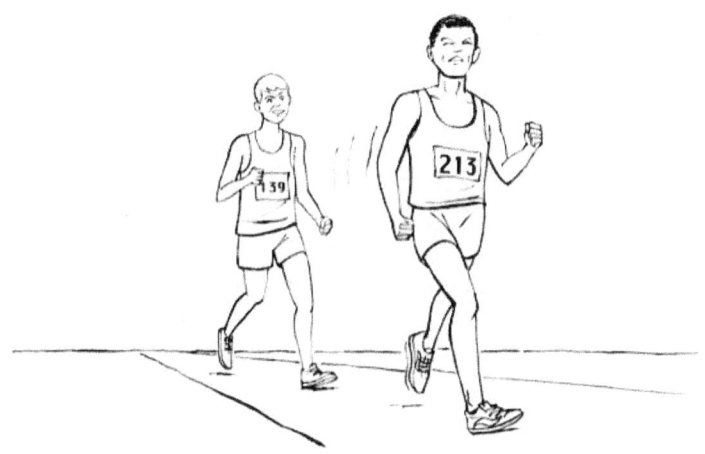

I had a good friend in the mid-west whom I ran several marathons with over the years. He was a good marathoner and usually ran a bit better times than I but not always. I liked this because it gave me an incentive to run a faster race each time we ran together. I felt that faster was better and would improve my finish times. That seemed to make sense and sometimes it did. However, one particular race proved that this idea can be folly. We had always been joking with each other as we ran. Just banter, good fun and no more. This one race though, Terry (not his real name), for whatever reason had a competitive streak going and just kept gradually increasing his pace. Maybe he was better prepared and just wanted to take advantage of that but, whatever the reason, I had to push a bit harder than I'd planned which was acceptable for a while but then it started to wear on me. In the end I had to pull back while he went ahead. He ran an excellent time but for me not so good. I ran rather slower than I expected.

Lesson: If your best friend in the world whom you would trust until death is running in the race beside you but intends to run that race faster than you, let him or her go. You're in the race to run your race not somebody else's.

#13 CHOOSE YOUR PATH

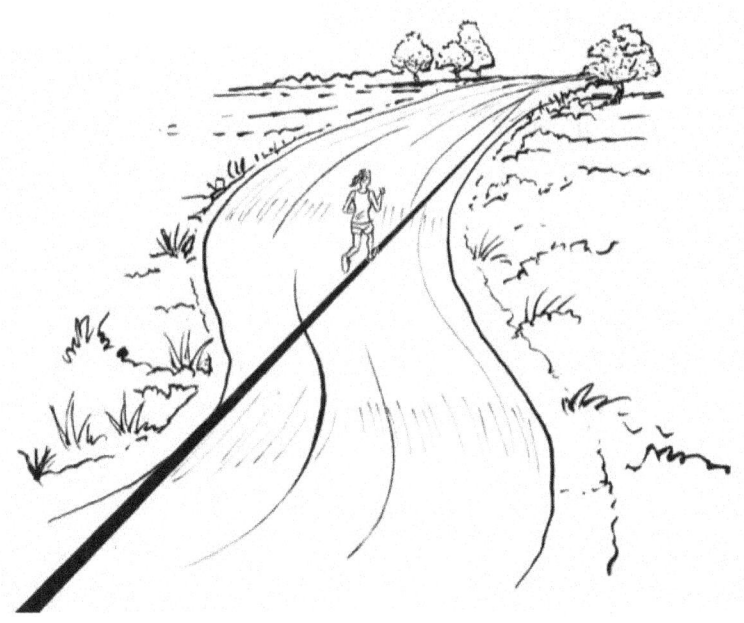

If you are running your very first marathon there are a lot of things you will learn. One of them is running the straightest course you can from start to finish. Some marathons make this really easy for you by putting a blue line on the road for you to follow which is the true 26 mile 385 yard distance. However, many don't so it's up to you to figure out the most direct route to the finish. This may seem like a trivial item but it's not, every stride counts. I ran one particular race (which I won't name since Athletic Directors get miffed about people mentioning disadvantages to their courses) which had a winding "S Pattern" for quite a few miles. I took the obvious shortest route by running "the tangents". That is by running a straight line from the apex of one bend to the apex of the next bend. You should do the same. Do NOT leave the assigned course by running on sidewalks or across restricted cones. That could give rise to accusations of course cutting which is something that will get you disqualified and thrown out of the race. Also, if you are aggressively running the tangents on a winding course you need to be aware of the other runners around you so as not to inhibit them in their races.

Lesson: Don't underestimate the effects of extra distance on your ability to reach the finish line faster. Always keep an eye on the road ahead. If you can save 2 yards on every bend in a winding course and there are 50 bends in your whole race (there are often many more) you've just saved 100 yards. There are 1,760 yards in a mile. If you are running an 8:00 mile (which is 480 seconds) for mile 26 the 100 yard improvement represents a 5.7% improvement in time (which is 27 seconds). You could change a 3 hour plus effort into a sub 3 hour result!

#14 KNOW YOUR PACE

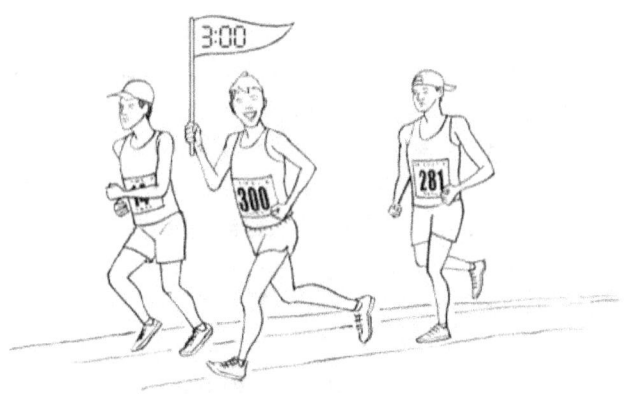

Despite spending many hours running in the weeks and months prior to a marathon surprisingly few marathoners, even experienced ones, seem to know exactly what pace they should set during their target race. There are various rules of thumb. **The first one** being "add 1 minute to your running economy pace at the start and gradually pick up the pace from there". You are already asking what is my "running economy" pace? Running economy is a measure of how much oxygen (or energy) your body requires to run at a particular pace. Since you should have run a number of races in preparation for your target marathon you should already know what your running economy pace is. **The second one** is to review the roadwork you have done in the months leading up to the race and compute a likely running schedule from it. What you do here is total the miles run for the ten weeks prior to the race (without including your taper) and divide that by ten. This gives you a weekly average. You then divide that number by seven to get a daily average. You then multiply that number by three. This number shows how far you can run before you collapse* if you are running at your training pace. Let's say the total miles you have run for the specified ten week period is 630 miles. This yields an average of 63 miles per week. Dividing that by seven gives a daily average of nine. When you multiply that by three you get 27. This means you can run the whole 26.22 miles of the marathon at your training pace and not fall away from it. **The third one** is split the race into three segments, run the first five miles slowly, run the next ten miles at increased pace and run the remaining 11.22 miles as best you feel you can. The more organized of these runners plan paces for the individual segments and hope they can maintain them. I will admit this is a bit vague but some runners do run their marathons to advantage this way.

Lesson: It's just plain common sense to have a pace plan for your marathon. Some marathons do help in this regard providing experienced marathoners who will run the marathon at a particular pace with a small banner showing what that pace is. However, not all marathons do this. So have a plan.

*As explained in the next Tip "collapse" only means a drastic fall off in pace.

#15 PLAN YOUR RACE AND RACE YOUR PLAN

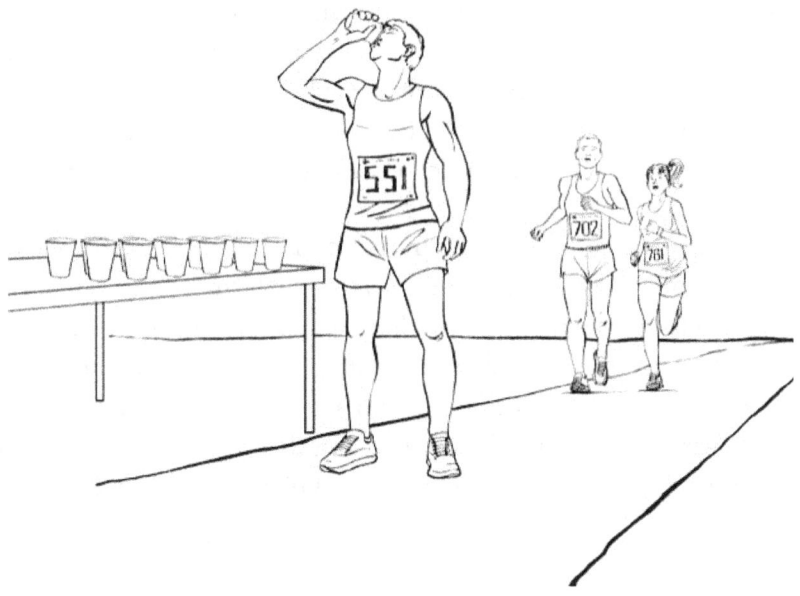

I have another running friend named Richard. He is a tall dude with a physically demanding job but he does have the body to match. Despite his height he is a rather good runner who can run sub-three hour marathons if he is well prepared. However, sometimes even though he's put in the miles and done them at the right pace he collapses on race day. I don't mean that he falls on the ground. No, nothing like that. What happens is his pace drops dramatically during the race and he goes from a 6:30 per mile pace down to 7:30 or even 8:00 minutes a mile and leaves a good race effort somewhere out on the course. Richard's problem is that he is an antsy kind of guy. He has difficulty taking it easy the week before the race. He gets distracted and doesn't sit down and prepare a race plan. Executing a good race plan includes not just training but (a) planning pace (b) being rested (c) planning nutrition and hydration. The odds of having a good result increase when all parts of the plan are executed. He also drinks beer to calm down which is very diuretic and draws much of the stored water out of his body. It was therefore no surprise to see him stopping frequently during races to drink water. The lack of planning and beer consumption affected his pace and his races. So even though he was often well prepared and could run the pace needed to get to the finish faster he often negated this obvious preparation in the days beforehand. He needed to run the race that he should have planned to run.

Lesson: As no other race the marathon is a preparation-oriented race. If your average milage is 45-50 miles or more for the 10-12 weeks prior to the race and you have done, at least, 2 or 3 training runs to 20 miles or more there is absolutely no reason you shouldn't finish the race comfortably <u>if you run at your training pace</u>. However, if you plan to run faster than that then you'd better be prepared to race at whatever that pace will be.

GUTS

#16 CONSEQUENCES

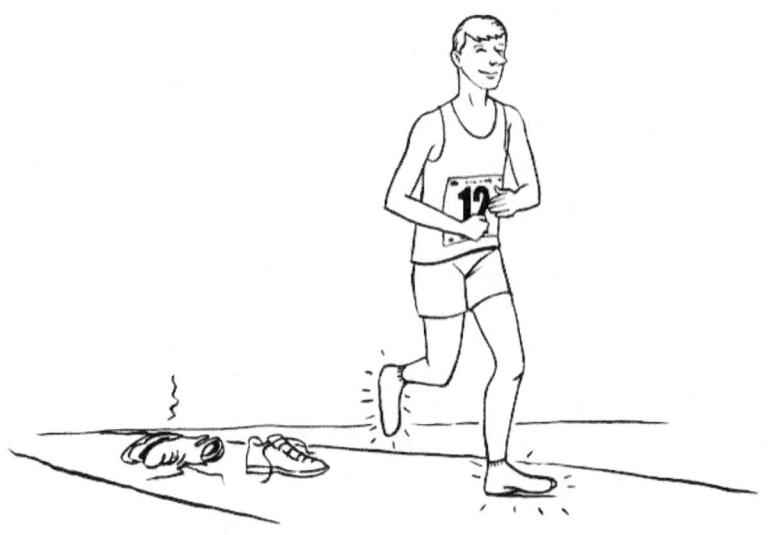

Despite the best preparation and a careful start sometimes things go wrong. You didn't get as much rest as you should have the week leading up to the race. Or, perhaps, despite some discussion with running pals who had already run the course it was proving much more challenging that you expected. For whatever reason, your best laid plans were going awry. It happens. At this point you need to keep a level head. Like much of life many seemingly insurmountable tasks are temporary, with enough grit and determination you will get through this latest challenge. So, chin up and face the music. I know a runner who was running an exceptional marathon until, at about 15 miles, one of his shoes simply collapsed. That's right it simply fell apart and he literally ran out of the shoe. He had chosen that pair of shoes because they were well broken in, had sufficient but not too many miles on them and looked perfectly fine for running this race. Yet one of them just died! Since he could not try to repair the collapsed shoe in some way and couldn't run in just the other one he did the only thing he could do. He ran without them! This is where smart preparation come into play. He was wearing the right kind of socks! He was running in Thorlos and they are extremely durable. He was an experienced marathoner with good form and excellent gait running on blacktop during the summer. The surface was benign enough that he covered the last 11.22 miles without too much bother. His feet were somewhat sore the next day but he recovered quickly. Best of all, he almost made his expected finish time.

Lesson: If you encounter an unexpected challenge during the race, don't panic. It may be just a temporary setback and you can recover. For instance, despite your best preparations, you felt that you had to walk at some point during your race. If this happens try to do it this way – run, jog, shuffle, walk. Then as you recover, regain your pace by reversing those steps – as in walk, shuffle, jog and then run.

#17 PREPARE, PREPARE, PREPARE

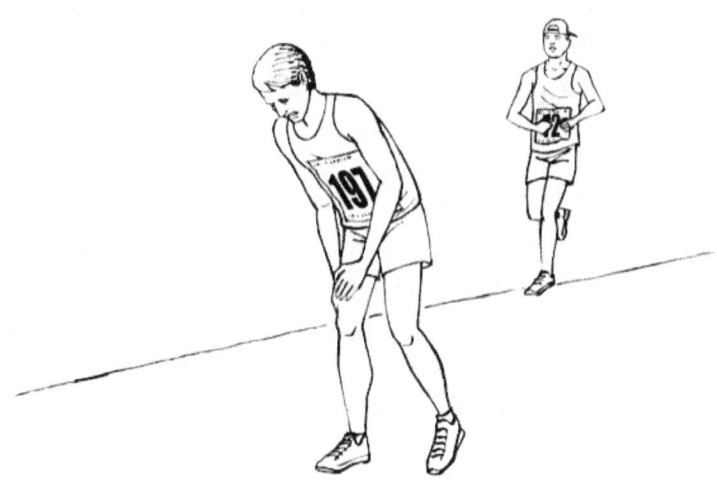

As no other race the marathon is all about preparation. Your performance on race day will be a direct function of the intelligent work you have done in the months and weeks leading up to your target race. I have a good friend named Peter who, after running many shorter races first, decided to move up to the marathon as his next big ambition. He was running a lot of milage already (averaging 60-70 miles per week and sometimes more) so he knew he had the basic road work done. He was also a really busy guy with a demanding engineering job which took up most of his time when he wasn't running. As a result, the length of time he had left to run became a key index in his busy life. He could spend an hour here, a half an hour there, but not the two or three hours he would need for long runs of 20 miles or more. So...he never did them! His longest "long run" before race day was to eleven miles. That's right – eleven miles! Even though he did everything else right and did as good a carbo load as anybody could have he started to "hit the wall" – you guessed it, at the half marathon point. That's right! Just halfway through the race he's already in trouble so it was a "death march" from there on. Despite hitting the half-marathon point in about 1:20 it took him a whole 2:35 to finish the second half! He was lucky to break four hours (much of it walking)! With enough long runs in his preparation, he could have easily taken an HOUR if not more off his finish time.

Lesson: If you have prepared properly, you'll be amazed at the number of people you will pass after Mile 20 who are barely moving. They will be doing what's called the "survival shuffle" – they either went out too fast or didn't prepare properly. You can smile quietly to yourself because you've done the right kind of work and will achieve your goal time for the race.

#18 GET YOUR PRIORITIES STRAIGHT

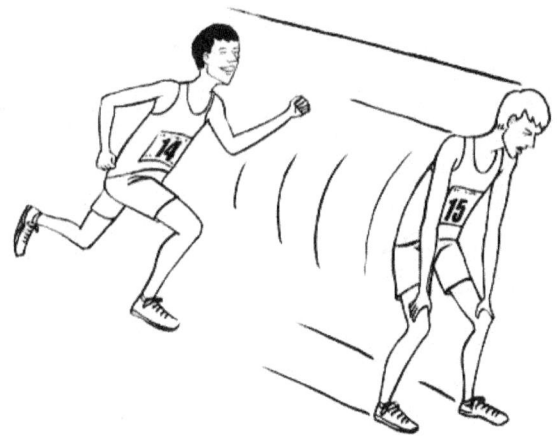

For many years I was a member of a mid-sized and accomplished Midwest running club. It had a wide cross section of runners of various capabilities both male and female. For a while, the club had a former East Coast university graduate who had run some good times for that school as a cross country athlete. However, he was always a short distance man never running much above 5K or 10K distances. Eventually, though, he decided to run a marathon as a new challenge. He prepared diligently and intelligently and I expected to hear that he had run a great time for his first race at the distance. It didn't happen. Despite his great preparation he decided the night before the race that he would try to break 2:30:00 for this first attempt in an effort to win the race. As a result, he started out running sub 6 minute miles. I know what you're thinking and I was thinking the same thing too as soon as I heard of it – "Really?". Yes, really. While he was perfectly capable of running those kinds of miles and much faster over a short distance in this case he was running a marathon. He kept this pace up until he got to about hallway but then things started to change. Apparently, glycogen depletion has set in early and it affected his pace, his stride and, perhaps, his common sense. He was determined to work through the change and continued apace. Somewhere past mile 20 he was slowed to almost a walk and eventually had to abandon the race and <u>was taken to the emergency room with severe dehydration</u>. He was lucky to recover fully after proper medical care and some days of rest.

Lesson: The marathon is a serious race. At all times during the race your goals for this major athletic endeavor should be, and remain, in this order.

(a) To finish the race
(b) To finish the race as comfortably as possible
(c) To finish the race in the best time possible for your capabilities

#19 OH! THOSE HILLS

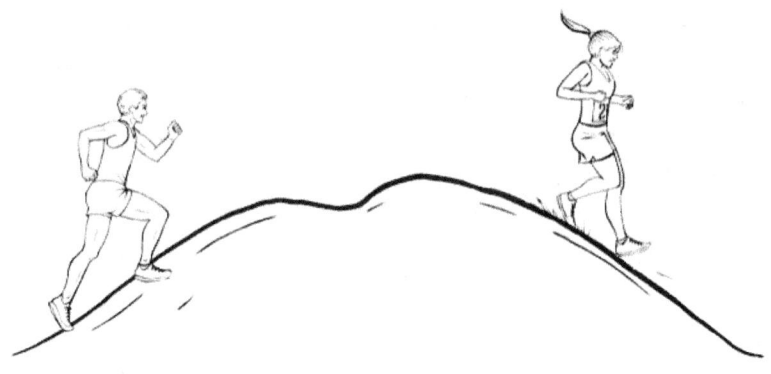

Anyone who's run the Boston Marathon knows about the Newton hills. Despite this, the course is still a net downhill. For some runners it can prove to be a fast course. However, it's not the only marathon run on a hilly course. In fact, some courses are run with hills as part of the featured terrain as an extra challenge. One that I will always remember is the City Of San Francisco Marathon. While it's highly advisable to seek a flat course if you want to run a fast time that doesn't mean you should avoid an otherwise great marathon just because it's got a few hills in it. Typically, runners lose about 4% of their effectiveness running uphill and may never regain it going downhill.

I always fancied myself as a good hill runner and, mostly, that was true. One thing I learned early on was to lean forward while running up the hill and then straighten up and increase my stride to maximize my pace while running down the hill. This proved to be an effective strategy. When initially addressing the hill, I would drop my hands down by my sides and angle my body into the hill to give me the best advantage. Then once I reached the top I would lengthen my stride as much as possible to regain as much of my lost momentum as I could.

Lesson: Don't be afraid of hills. They can be to your advantage at times. After many miles of running at a fixed gait you can become cramp-prone. Running the odd hill here and there will change your stride significantly and may ward off the possibility of cramping. No matter how good a runner you are, you will lose a few percent of your effort to the hill.

#20 THE END OF YOUR TETHER

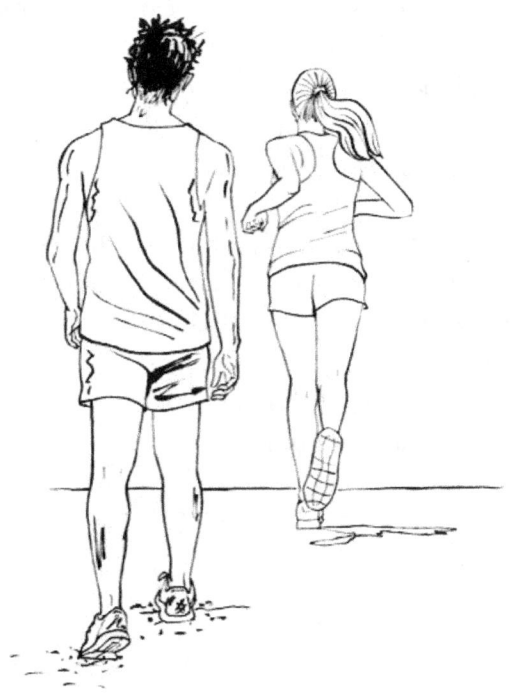

I've left this until to the end because it's something you may not want to think about before your race starts but…despite your best planning, your best preparation and everything else going right – it may not be your day. You may get to a point past 20 miles, maybe, when you think you just can't go any farther. I know it's happened to me. It's happened to many average runners. Whether you've "hit the wall" really hard and "bonked" to a high degree or just been overcome by the sheer monotony of putting one foot in front of the other at a slower and slower pace you've gotten to a point where you think you just can't go any further. Take heart! It's only a race and nobody's really expecting great things of you except yourself. This part of the event is where character is tested – and revealed. Simply stop and start walking. If you're beyond 20 miles there's 10kM or less to the finish. The average walker can cover a mile in 20 minutes. You're a trained runner, you will get there faster. If you're at 21 miles you can feasibly reach the finish in 75 minutes walking. However, you're a fit and well prepared runner. Energy will return and much sooner than you think. Remember the routine from Tip #16 – walk, shuffle, jog and then run. Before you know it you'll be running again? How about that!

Lesson: Unless threatened by injury or illness (e.g., heatstroke) don't ever give up on your race – no matter how hard it seems to go on and how easy it seems to quit. Don't be ashamed if you have to walk. Even in a totally "walled out" state, as a well prepared runner, you can walk a mile in 15 minutes. If you're at mile 22 you can still finish the race in an hour or less.